When You Know You're Dying

*12 Thoughts to Guide You
Through the Days Ahead*

James E. Miller

Willowgreen Publishing

To Holly, Chris, Martha, Carrie, and John,
loved ones all

This book would not have come to be without Holly Book, Chris Crawford, Martha Ebel, Carrie Hackney, and John Saynor. These five shared their experiences, offered their ideas, made numerous editorial suggestions, and left their very distinctive imprints on this work. I am extremely grateful to them all. Clare Barton proofed the text. Marty Herman executed the drawings and consulted about the overall design. Just Sue Graphic Design handled the layout. And my wife, Bernie, was ever present and ever helpful, as always.

Willowgreen Publishing
PO Box 25180
Fort Wayne, Indiana 46825
219/424-7916

Library of Congress Catalogue
Card Number: 97-60133

ISBN 1-885933-24-X

Teach me your mood, O patient stars!
Who climb each night the ancient sky,
Leaving in space no shade, no scars,
No trace of age, no fear to die.

RALPH WALDO EMERSON

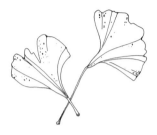

For the thing that I fear comes upon me,
and what I dread befalls me.
I am not at ease, nor am I quiet.

THE BOOK OF JOB

Dear God, be good to me.
The sea is so wide,
and my boat is so small.

BRETON FISHERMAN'S PRAYER

What was once unimaginable to you must now be imagined. What once seemed strange and awful—what may *still* seem strange and awful—must now be given its place in your life. In one way or another, you've been told you are dying.

Perhaps you've known that for quite some time and you're no longer surprised. Or perhaps you've learned it only recently and it's still a terrible shock. Either way, you're in unknown territory now. You haven't done this before. Those who love you are probably as unsteady and unsure as you. And the larger world around you, with a few important exceptions, will not make this time much easier for you.

Our culture does not handle dying very well. It's no longer a part of our everyday lives as it was for our ancestors. We don't look upon it as directly as they did. We don't live with it as closely. Most of us don't participate in it as personally. So when the news comes that we're dying, we're at a definite loss. We have so little background for knowing what to do. It all seems so unfamiliar and frightening. This can be a very upsetting time for everyone.

If you're like most people, you don't have much energy to spare right now. For that reason I've written this book so you can read it fairly easily. The words are direct, the ideas are simple, and the chapters are short. At the same time, I believe there's value in taking your time as you enter this period of your life and as you ponder what all this means for you. So I've included a number of quotations from

To begin depriving death its greatest advantage over us,
let us adopt a way contrary to that common one;
let us deprive death of its strangeness,
let us frequent it, let us get used to it.

MICHEL DE MONTAIGNE

If you want to die happily, learn to live.
If you want to live happily, learn to die.

LATIN PROVERB

many different people for you to reflect upon. A number of these quotations were composed by women and men who were themselves dying.

I've done one more thing in preparing this book for you: I've spent a lot of time with five individuals who either work or have worked daily with dying people. So in addition to my own experiences as a clergyperson, counselor, and family member, I've drawn upon the wisdom and expertise of some of the most knowledgeable, compassionate people I know. If you find the words of this book helpful, remember that Carrie, Martha, Chris, John, and Holly are behind them every bit as much as I. And remember that all of us are behind you and want the best for you. That's why we've done what we've done. ◪

Jim Miller

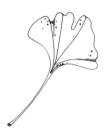

Nature never repeats herself,
and the possibilities of one human soul
will never be found in another.

ELIZABETH CADY STANTON

For an impenetrable shield,
stand inside yourself.

HENRY DAVID THOREAU

To be what we are,
and to become what we are capable of becoming,
is the only end of life.

ROBERT LOUIS STEVENSON

1

Be who you are.

Traumatic news has rocked your life: your days on earth are limited. You've always known that, of course. Everyone does. You've been aware that anyone who is born must one day die. But now the truth strikes home in a way you've never realized. This is not about just anyone—it's about you.

As you work through all this means for you, and for those around you, it's important to keep one fundamental fact in mind. While a monumental change has occurred in your life, one thing has not changed at all: who you are. You're the same person you've always been. You have the same personality, the same idiosyncrasies, the same likes and dislikes, the same memories. You are still you, and you dare not forget that.

• *You are uniquely, unrepeatably you.* There is no one exactly like you. There never has been, never will be. That means, among other things, that you'll go through this experience now in your own original way. You will not conform to some rigid pattern because none exists for you. You will create your own. The best way for you to go through this time is in the way that's true for you. How will you know? You'll learn by doing. You'll make your way by going.

• *You are more than your illness.* A disease has taken center stage in your life. Your doctors study it, measure it, treat it, and talk about it. Sometimes you may understand all this, and sometimes not. Family and friends will often want to know the details of what's happening to you, and how you're feeling, and what they can do for you. Your sickness may begin to feel like a deficiency or a flaw. You

I'll walk where my own nature would be leading;
it vexes me to choose another guide.

EMILY BRONTË

Be at peace with your own soul.
Enter eagerly into the treasure house
that is inside you.
The ladder leading to the Kingdom
is hidden within your soul.
Dive into yourself, and in your soul
you will discover the stairs by which to ascend.

ISAAC OF NINEVAH

may be treated only as a patient, or worse, as an invalid. But the truth is clear: your disease does not define you. Your identity remains apart from your illness. Cling to that knowledge. From time to time, you may need to remind others as well.

• *You are more than your body.* It's common for others to concentrate on what's happening to you physically. You may do that yourself. These internal and external changes to your body can be uncomfortable, unpleasant, even distressing. But the person you are physically is only one part of who you are really. It is your mind, your heart, and your soul that complete you and make you a whole. During this time of your life, in fact, these other, less visible parts of you may become more important than the visible.

• *You're who you <u>know</u> you are, not who others <u>think</u> you are.* You may find that people expect you to be somehow different because you're dying. They may treat you differently, either consciously or unconsciously. However it happens, they're acting this way for themselves, not for you. By emphasizing the differences between you and them, they hide from the one important thing you share in common—one day they, like you, will also die. You don't have to like the way they treat you, but it will help if you can understand why they're doing it. After all, until recently you may have done the same thing to someone else. For the time at hand, be clear about who you are within yourself. Hold fast to that essence that is yours alone.

As you proceed through this period of your life, just be you. Keep being you. And day by day, determine to become more and more that person you're being invited to be. No one can do this but you. And no one can do it any better than you. ◪

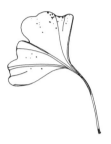

Seeing is believing,
but feeling is God's own truth.

IRISH PROVERB

Below the surface-stream, shallow and light,
Of what we say we feel—below the stream,
A light, of what we think we feel—there flows
With noiseless current strong, obscure, and deep,
The central stream of what we feel indeed.

MATTHEW ARNOLD

2

Feel any and all of your feelings.

You have never done what you're about to do. You have not gone where you're about to go. As you enter this strange and unfamiliar territory, it will help to remember five facts about your reactions.

• *You will have many feelings.* You may feel unspeakably sad about your situation. You may fear what will happen before you die, as you die, or after you die. You may be afraid of pain, or disfigurement, or abandonment. You may become listless and depressed. At one time or another you may feel shocked or confused, anxious or panicky, helpless or lonely. You may feel hurt, or angry, or even enraged. You may feel guilty or ashamed about what you've done or not done. You may be envious of others. As time goes by, many other feelings may surface: relief, love, wonder, pride, even joy. You will not necessarily have all these feelings, but you'll certainly have some of them. And sometimes you may have none of them—it will seem you're without feelings. It happens.

• *Your feelings will be unpredictable.* There will be no order to your emotions. They'll come and go when they want, and where they want, and how they want. They may appear one at a time, or they may erupt in a jumble, sometimes even contradicting one another. They may pass quickly or slowly, softly or loudly, easily or painfully. They may surprise you, popping up when you least anticipate them. That's the nature of feelings.

• *Your feelings are likely to be intense.* It's all relative: what's intense for one person may seem subdued to another. But however strong your emotions have been in the past, they're likely to be

Rich tears!
What power lies in those falling drops.
MARY DELARIVIER MANLEY

You are healed of a suffering
only by experiencing it to the full.
MARCEL PROUST

stronger now. This can be a chaotic time for you. The pressures can feel enormous. The possibilities can seem frightening. Under these circumstances, unexpectedly powerful emotions are to be expected.

• *You will grieve.* Anytime a person loses or is deprived of something or someone important, it's both natural and healthy to mourn. The losses you now face are immense. They include your health, your work, the roles you've grown accustomed to, all the plans you've made, various dreams you've held. You will have to relinquish your security, your home, your family, your relationships. Eventually you'll have to let go of physical life itself. All this will take great energy on your part, and it will tire you. But, in time, your grieving will also help free you. And it will help free others too.

• *You have permission to feel whatever you feel.* Some people may try to tell you the opposite. Verbally or nonverbally, they may ask you to hide or deny your feelings. They may tell you "Be strong!" when what they're really saying is "Please don't cry!". Let's face it—it is difficult to be around someone in deep pain. Perhaps that awareness can help you put aside any messages from others about restricting your feelings. Look for the permission you deserve from those who really understand you, perhaps those who have been around dying people before. The best permission to feel comes from an undisputed authority: yourself.

Always remember: your feelings are neither right nor wrong. They are a sign that you care deeply, that you value life and love, and that you are taking seriously what is happening to you. As long as your feelings are honest, they're valid. And so are you. ◪

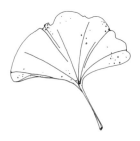

What soap is for the body,
tears are for the soul.

JEWISH PROVERB

Give sorrow words; the grief that does not speak
Whispers the oe'r fraught heart and bids it break.

WILLIAM SHAKESPEARE

It takes two to speak the truth—
one to speak, and another to hear.

HENRY DAVID THOREAU

3

Let your feelings out.

Right now it's not easy to feel all your emotions. The pain and sorrow can go very deep. The way your feelings may sometimes overpower you can be disconcerting, if not alarming. But if you can give your feelings room, you'll find they will lead you where you need to go. One direction they'll often lead you is toward their expression.

You needn't vent all your emotions. You may not want to or be able to. But you will do well to channel various feelings into some form of communication. Afterwards you'll feel a sense of release and perhaps a calm. You may see things in new ways. You may draw closer to others and they to you. You may learn lessons that surprise you and affirm you.

• *Let out your feelings to the one who really matters: yourself.* You don't even have to use language. A good cry can express what you feel as completely as any words. You may wish to write about what's going on inside. If that's the case, you might keep a journal, or pen your feelings into poems, or compose your autobiography. These can all be a way to record your personal growth, as well as a legacy you can pass on. Other dying people have channeled their feelings into drawing and sculpting, quilting and woodworking, music and dance. Anything that has helped you express yourself in the past can help you now. But you can also branch out and try an expression that's entirely new. What's stopping you?

• *Honor your feelings by speaking them to another person.* More than any other time in your life, you need and deserve the interest and concern of someone who cares. Find someone who's a good lis-

He speaketh not; and yet there lies
A conversation in his eyes.
HENRY WADSWORTH LONGFELLOW

The best prayers often have more groans than words.
JOHN BUNYAN

Out of the deep I have called to you, O Lord:
Lord, hear my voice.
PSALM 130

tener and talk about what's important to you. Trust your instincts and you'll figure out who can be open to what you have to say. It's often especially meaningful when that person can be someone you've long known and loved. Sometimes, however, those people aren't able to hear all you have to say just yet—it's all too hard, too much, too soon. Perhaps then someone who has less at stake can be a better listener for you. You may choose to turn to a chaplain or clergyperson, a counselor or social worker, a nurse or doctor. Have you met someone from your area hospice yet? You'll find these people are usually very understanding, for they've been around dying people many times before. More than that, they like being around you—that's why they keep doing what they do.

• *Another option is to release your feelings in a group setting.* Some communities have support groups for those who know they're dying. Check with your local hospice, hospital, or home care agency. Or try your area cancer society, heart association, or AIDS task force. Perhaps your family members, friends, and colleagues can become your support group. Nowadays groups even meet on the internet.

• *Finally, you can express yourself, not just to others, but to The Supreme Other.* If you're so inclined, you can pray your feelings, just as people have done for ages. You might want to try a few of the Psalms to see if some of those deep-felt prayers don't capture some of your own emotions. Your feelings can also find a welcome home as you meditate or worship.

However you choose to do it, allow the energy of your emotions to flow over you and through you and on beyond you. Only then can you begin to experience a sense of peace in the midst of the confusion.◪

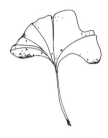

We want people to feel with us
more than act for us.
GEORGE ELIOT (MARY ANN EVANS)

Let those who have need of more
ask for it humbly.
And let those who have need of less
thank God.
SAINT BENEDICT

4

Make your needs and wants known.

Chances are good you'll be reluctant to follow this guideline. You've been told through the years you shouldn't be "overly dependent." You've been exposed to suggestions about "paddling your own canoe" and "standing on your own two feet." That's what happens in a culture like ours that promotes rugged individualism and sturdy independence. Consequently, you may hesitate to inconvenience other people. You may feel it's selfish to be so clear about what you need from those around you.

It may take special effort to allow yourself to depend on others. But that's one of the tasks before you. The job is too big to do all by yourself. And despite what you may have learned, there's nothing weak or shameful about accepting assistance. From time to time, everyone needs a helping hand.

• *You'll have various needs and wants.* Because you're a whole human being, you have a whole set of drives and desires. Some are physical, having to do with your personal care and comfort, and even your survival. Some needs are emotional, relating to your mental well-being and growth. You have social needs, seen both in your desire for company and in your wish to be alone at times. You have spiritual needs, too, whatever form these may take in your life, and environmental needs, relating to the surroundings you're in and how those surroundings are equipped and arranged.

• *Your needs and wants will change.* What you desire today, you may not tomorrow. The assistance you need at the moment will not be the same assistance you'll need weeks or months from now. Flexibility will be key for you and those near you.

Shared joy is double joy
and shared sorrow is half-sorrow.
SWEDISH PROVERB

The fragrance always remains
in the hand that gives the rose.
MAHATMA GANDHI

• *Others will not automatically know what you need.* They've never been exactly where you are. They're not you. Since they cannot read your mind, you must tell them. The best way to communicate is simply, directly, and honestly. They'll need your guidance if they're to provide the right assistance. Otherwise they'll be frustrated in their attempts. Begin developing a list of your needs and wants, then keep it handy. When someone says "Let me know if there's anything I can do," let them know.

• *Your helpers have their own needs and limits.* Some are good at supporting you psychologically and others are better at doing that by cooking or cleaning or running errands for you. Some are ready to speak frankly with you, others are great at making you laugh, and still others would prefer to discuss the weather. When you ask a favor, keep in mind who you're asking and what they're good at.

• *In meeting your needs, others can meet <u>their</u> needs.* You're not the only one who feels helpless. Those who love you wish this wasn't happening to you. They wish they could change it, knowing they cannot. But at least they can do little things to help out and show they care. They feel like they're contributing somehow and they're not so powerless.

• *You may want and need an advocate.* In time it may become tiring to handle all this communication. You may wish to select a person to speak for you. Whether they're a family member, a friend, or a professional, they can run interference for you and help preserve your energy.

By letting your needs and wants be known, you're making it possible for a true sense of community to develop. This may not have been your intention, but it can be a wonderful opportunity for everyone involved. ◪

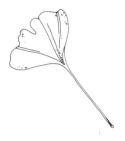

Good company is a good coach.

JOHN CLARKE

It brings comfort and encouragement
to have companions in whatever happens.

DIO CHRYSOTOM

We are all travelers
in the wilderness of this world,
and the best we can find in our travels
is an honest friend.

ROBERT LOUIS STEVENSON

5

Let whoever is close to you take this journey with you.

The road before you is not one you wish to take. But you were not given a choice. And now this is a road no one else can take for you, no matter who they are, no matter how much they love you. But you need not travel alone. You can travel together, you and those close to you.

Who are these people? Only you can know. They may be members of your family, those who have loved you from the start and have made with you a place called home. Or these people may be family in a larger sense—family of the heart. They may be bonded to you, not legally, but emotionally and spiritually. It's a bond that can be every bit as secure and loving and rewarding.

How many are these people? Only you can say. We all differ in how many we let get close to us and how close we let them get. Maybe your inner circle will have room for just one or two people. Or maybe you'll want to include quite a few. There will be a limit, however, to the number you choose—you dare not spread yourself too thin. Time is limited. So is energy.

Why should you journey together?

• *You need others.* Your journey is demanding. The way can be long. For those times when you're lonely, you could use a reassuring touch. When you're afraid, you could stand a comforting embrace. When you're feeling down, you might appreciate a sign that someone cares. If you're not sure you can go on, you can be reminded how you've persevered before and where your strength lies today. When

After you had taken your leave,
I found God's footprints on my floor.

RABINDRANATH TAGORE

Bless to me, O God, the earth beneath my feet,
Bless to me, O God, the path whereon I go,
Bless to me, O God, the people whom I meet,
Today, tonight, and tomorrow.

CELTIC BLESSING

you try to make sense of what has happened, someone you trust can help you sort through your questions and be a witness to your answers. When you need a confirmation that your life has mattered and you will not be forgotten, someone you love can bestow that blessing on you. These are things you cannot easily do for yourself, but others can do them for you. And often they want to do them.

• *Others need you.* Time is also short for those who love you. They want to make the most of whatever time is left. Perhaps there are things they haven't said to you, or things they want to say again. Maybe there are situations they want to rectify, or memories they want to rehearse, or feelings they want to share.

Just as you have losses to grieve, so do they. There is much they'll miss, and some things they're already missing. By acknowledging their feelings and mourning what they're losing, they can prepare for what lies before them. The time ahead will still be painful, but they will have begun the grieving process with you rather than apart from you. That can lessen any potential complications and minimize any lingering regrets.

• *Together you can make this the journey of a lifetime.* You can live the moments you share in whichever ways you choose. You can fill them with whatever gives you pleasure and meaning. You can use them for whatever deepens your connection and closeness. You can open yourselves to the mystery that surrounds you and approach it hand-in-hand with appreciation and awe. You can make your days count as only the two of you, or the group of you, know how.

Just remember: you're all in this together. And however you're related, you're now family. ◪

27

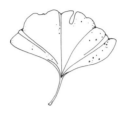

Life is either a daring adventure,
or nothing.

HELEN KELLER

Of all paths a man could strike into,
there is, at any given moment,
a best path which, here and now,
it were of all things wisest for him to do.
To find this path, and walk in it,
is the one thing needful for him.

THOMAS CARLYLE

6

Assert your right to make
your own decisions.

One person's voice deserves to be heard above all others—yours.
You have more at stake than anyone. So this is not a time to try to
please everyone or to live up to others' expectations. It's a time to be
true, above all, to yourself. It's a time to take control of your own
decisionmaking as much as you're able.

• *Make your own lifestyle decisions.* Like everyone, you have limits as to time and money and energy. Admittedly, you don't live in a
vacuum—you must also take other people's lives into account. But
you're the one who has the right, within reason, to call the shots
now. How do you want to spend the time that's left? Will you con-
tinue to work? Will you spend your days as usual, or will you do
something different? Will you travel, or will you stay home? Who
will be around you?

This can be an unusually freeing time for you. You may choose to
do what you've always wanted but never allowed yourself to do. You
may let go of some of the unnecessary "shoulds" in your life. You
may come into the open in a way that finally feels natural and real.
Odd as it may sound, you may begin to truly live.

• *Make your own medical decisions.* This can be a formidable task.
You may struggle to understand all the jargon, procedures, technol-
ogy, and options. You'll want to work with healthcare professionals
who communicate well. You may wish to obtain second and third
opinions from physicians, or consult with other people whose wisdom you trust, or read as much as you can about your disease and

Do not be too timid
or squeamish about your actions.
All life is an experiment.

RALPH WALDO EMERSON

Risk! Risk anything!
Care no more for the opinions of others.
Do the hardest thing on earth for you.
Act for yourself. Face the truth.

KATHERINE MANSFIELD
(nearing her own death)

prognosis. Ultimately though, it will be up to you to determine the course of your own medical care. You can decide which treatments you'll pursue and which you'll forgo. You can decide where you'll receive care, what kind, how often, and for how long.

• *Make your own end-of-life decisions.* Only you will know when you're ready to do this, but it's extremely important you do it while you're still alert. Some of these decisions will enhance your own comfort and peace of mind. Other decisions will help those who survive you. Those who love you will have the satisfaction of knowing they're following your wishes. There'll be less confusion at the end.

It's important to make decisions regarding all your financial matters, which can create various advantages for you and your loved ones. You may want to determine how your personal possessions will be distributed. If you haven't already, execute a will. Otherwise the government will decide what happens to your estate, and your ideas are more fitting than theirs. It will also help to communicate your wishes about the disposition of your body and your thoughts about your funeral or memorial service.

It's important to execute advance medical directives, including a living will, spelling out which life-sustaining measures you do and do not wish to have taken in a medical emergency. Notarized copies of these directives should be given to your physicians, the hospital, and close family members. Consult an attorney about other documents you can have drawn up which will name who can make various medical and legal decisions for you, should you become unable.

Clearly, you have many decisions to make. Some will come naturally and easily, and others may take a great deal of effort. But by taking control of these decisions now, you'll come to feel more at ease with what lies ahead. So will those who love you. ◪

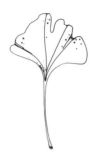

A day is lost if one has not laughed.

FRENCH PROVERB

A life without festivities
is a long road without inns.

DEMOCRITUS

Come, let us give a little time to folly,
and even in a melancholy day,
let us find time for an hour of pleasure.

SAINT BONAVENTURA

7

Embrace that which promotes your well-being and growth.

Now is not the time to delay your satisfactions. It's the time to live life to the full. What might that mean for you? The following questions will help you know.

• *What makes you happy?* What do you always look forward to? What gives you such satisfaction that time flies while you're doing it? A hobby, a craft, a passion, a labor of love? It may be something you've always done, or something you've always *wanted* to do. Perhaps it's a dear one you enjoy being with, or several dear ones. Maybe it involves a special treat. Whatever gives you pleasure, give it prominence.

• *What soothes you?* What calms and relaxes you? Some like quiet music and others prefer quiet all by itself. You may be soothed by prayer, by guided visualization, or by inspiring quotations. Maybe you'd like something read to you or sung for you. A pleasant daily routine might help you unwind gently, perhaps as evening approaches or as nighttime falls. Look for those things that give you serenity and then draw them close.

• *What energizes you?* At times you may want to feel invigorated. What adds a sparkle to your life? What gives you zest? Sometimes expending energy will give you more energy, especially if it comes from your heart or soul. Other people can also enliven you with their spirit and spunk.

• *What makes you laugh?* However heavy this time may be, it doesn't have to be only that way. People in your situation have often been heard to say, "I didn't expect to laugh as much as I do." That may

Die when I may,
I want it said of me by those who knew me best,
that I always plucked a thistle and planted a flower
where I thought a flower would grow.

ABRAHAM LINCOLN

I rejoice in life for its own sake.
Life is no brief candle to me.
It is a sort of splendid torch which
I have got hold of for the moment,
and I want to make it burn as brightly as possible
before handing it on to future generations.

GEORGE BERNARD SHAW

sound odd to you at the moment, but one day you may say the same thing. It's not only fun to laugh—it's therapeutic. It helps your body release its natural painkillers and healing agents. So go ahead: joke with people and invite them to joke with you. Make time for whatever gives you a chuckle.

• *What nourishes you?* What helps you feel healthier and more whole? What strengthens you and helps you flourish? Perhaps art feeds you. Or literature. Or good conversation. Perhaps what nurtures you is being in nature or having nature brought in to you. You'll know by now some individuals are more nourishing than others. Gather around you whatever or whoever gives you sustenance, then feast.

• *What gives your days meaning?* Is it the impact others are having on your life, or the impact you're making on others, or is it both? Is it what you're learning, or what you're teaching, or is it neither? Do you find purpose in what you do or simply in who you are? Meaning can be difficult to define but you know it when it appears. Such moments feel rich and full, and your life has substance and value. When you come upon these experiences, treasure them.

• *What inspires you?* What offers you hope and gives you courage? What motivates you to go on? Some people find it in their faith and some in their fellowship. Some discover it in the lives of others and some in their own stories. Inspiration cannot be manufactured—it can only be recognized and then captured. Each time you see it coming, grab hold of it.

• *Who loves you?* Who basks in your presence? Who draws out your better self? Who cherishes their time with you? And who do you cherish being with? Whatever you do with the time you have left, do this: love, and allow yourself to be loved. Life may be limited, but love doesn't have to be. ◨

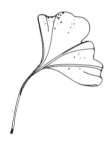

Remember that you have only one soul;
that you have only one death to die;
that you have only one life,
which is short and has to be lived by you alone;
and there is only one glory, which is eternal.
If you do this, there will be many things
about which you care nothing.

Teresa of Avila

8

Let go of that which blocks your well-being and growth.

As you move toward those experiences that are positive and freeing, you may choose to move away from those with the opposite effect. You must determine for yourself what is best here, although it may help to talk this over with someone you respect. The following thoughts may also assist you.

• *To "let go" will mean different things depending on what's blocking you.* This doesn't necessarily mean "get rid of," but in some cases that's exactly what you may strive to do, and with good reason. Discarding a bad habit or a destructive behavior will be both a wise decision and a mature step forward. To let go can also mean to limit an influence upon you, or to release yourself from an unnecessary obligation, or to put something behind you that is best forgotten.

• *Some blocks may be within you.* You may be carrying unhealthy ideas about the kind of person you are, or the kind of treatment you deserve, or the kind of future you can expect. These thoughts may have started very early in your life. They may be so ingrained you don't even realize they're there. Suddenly, knowing what you now know, the blinders may begin to fall away. Some of the limits you've learned to live with may have kept you away from other people. If you want to change and if you want your life to improve, what better reason is there than this and what better time than now?

• *Some blocks may be in others.* Certain people may drag you down. For whatever reason, they may be embittered or belittling or downright hostile. They may try to make decisions for you or hold

We must, strictly speaking,
at every moment give each other up
and let each other go
and not hold each other back.

RAINIER MARIA RILKE

May I tell you
why it seems to me a good thing
for us to remember wrong
that has been done to us?
That we may forgive it.

CHARLES DICKENS

out unfair expectations of you. You dare not allow such people to ruin this time. Something needs to be said to them in an understanding yet firm way, either by you or your chosen advocate. Perhaps that will be enough. Or perhaps your only solution will be to remove yourself from the presence of such people. These can be ticklish situations, but they must be addressed if you're to have the comfortable and wholesome environment you're entitled to.

• *If you spend this time protecting others, you'll endanger yourself.* It's dangerous for you to try to take care of everyone else's feelings and needs. In fact, it's more than dangerous—it's impossible. You cannot make everything right for everybody. Those close to you will have their own problems and concerns. You cannot take those away from them, anymore than they can take yours away from you. But you can suggest that each of you be responsible with your own concerns, thoughts, and feelings, and then you can follow your own suggestion. Rather than spend your energy protecting each other, you can invest it supporting and appreciating one another. Not only is that healthier for all of you, but it's a lot more enjoyable.

• *This is a perfect time for forgiveness.* Do you wish to ask another's pardon for something you've done? Now is an excellent time. Do you wish to forgive someone for what they've done to you? This is an ideal moment in both your lives. Do you need your own forgiveness? Find a way to give and receive that so you can live these days more at peace. Perhaps this whole issue of forgiveness is connected to your relationship with God. Are you searching for a divine pardon? Or does it work the other way—do you feel you need to make peace with God about what has been done to you? Whatever has happened in your life, forgiveness is possible.◪

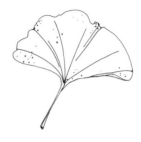

What was hard to bear is sweet to remember.

PORTUGUESE PROVERB

A good story is medicine to my bones.

ABRAHAM LINCOLN

Some memories are realities,
and are better than anything
that can ever happen to me again.

WILLA CATHER

9

Tell your story.

Your life has been a drama. There have been high points and low points, periods of excitement and strange twists of fate. Once you begin to tell your tale, you may surprise yourself with all that has happened to you. And you may be surprised at the interest others will show in your story. You know things no one else knows. You remember things others have long forgotten. Now is a wonderful time to share what is yours, so that it can become more than yours.

• *You can reminisce.* A good way to begin is simply to start talking. What memories stand out? What are your earliest recollections? Your favorite ones? Your saddest? Your funniest? Weave in the stories of your ancestors and other family members. Leaf through newspaper clippings, letters you've saved, old pictures you've collected, and see what pops into your mind.

You've spent your whole life preparing this tale. Tell it now with flair. Throw in those details that add spice and life. Imitate people's voices. Rouse your listeners' curiosity and keep them guessing while you spin your yarn. Invite people's questions and then lean back and paint a picture in words.

• *You can preserve your memories.* Telling your stories to others is one way of preserving them, but you may prefer a more permanent method. They may too. Are you a writer? Save your stories in a journal or notebook. Are you an organizer? Build a scrapbook with pictures and keepsakes. Are you an historian? Produce a biographical remembrance. You might even have it published, if only for family members. Do you like genealogy? Build your family tree.

Childhood has no forebodings,
but then it is soothed by no memories
of outlived sorrow.
GEORGE ELIOT (MARY ANN EVANS)

I shall remember while the light lives yet
And in the night time I shall not forget.
ALGERNON CHARLES SWINBURNE

Do the work of preserving the story yourself or invite others to join you. Tell your tales into a tape recorder with others present if you wish. Allow yourself to be interviewed on videotape. You could even ask others to add their memories to yours so it becomes a community project. This need not be a one-time event—it can stretch over weeks and months.

• *You can organize and share your thoughts.* You have more to pass on than just what you remember. You also have what you think and feel. Have you ever taken the time to spell out your ideas about topics that interest you and others? What goes into your philosophy of life? What are your beliefs? In your eyes, what are life's most important lessons? What would you do differently if you had it to do over? What would you never change? What would you like your grandchildren to know about you? What message do you want to leave them?

If all this sounds like too much work right now, remember you can tell your story in very quiet ways too. Sometimes those are the best stories of all. All it takes is two willing souls, two grateful hearts, one quiet room, and a few open hours here and there. You'll not only *recall* memories—you'll *make* memories.

However you choose to tell your story, never doubt it has value to others. It's one way you'll be remembered. It's another way you'll be loved. And it's an important way you can leave your mark, for your tale will intertwine with all the others through the ages. ◪

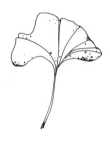

Dost thou love life?
Then do not squander time,
for that's the stuff life is made of.
BENJAMIN FRANKLIN

Do you know that disease and death
must needs overtake us, no matter what we are doing?
What do you wish to be doing when it overtakes you?
If you have anything better to be doing
when you are so overtaken, get to work on that.
EPICTETUS

10

Decide what you yet want to do, then do it.

You've probably asked yourself this question as a mental exercise before: "What would I do if I had only weeks or months to live?" That question is no longer theoretical. It's real—extremely real. What will you do with the days you're now given?

Is there something you've put off doing, thinking there would always be time? Have you been carrying a dream, one you'd now like to help come true? Are there places you want to go for the first time, or the last? Do you want to leave a legacy that will survive you?

Perhaps your goals are internal. Do you wish to turn your attention to fighting your illness, or perhaps accepting it? Do you want to deepen yourself spiritually or perhaps open yourself emotionally? Are you ready to love yourself more, or perhaps blame others less?

Maybe you're not inclined toward much change at all. Maybe you simply want to keep doing what you've always done for as long as you can. And maybe what you want to do is simply learn how to relax and begin letting go.

Whatever you wish to do with this time, here are a few suggestions for making the most of it:

• *Be clear about what you want to do.* That's the only way you can be sure you're claiming this time as your own. Write your ideas down if it helps, or speak them to someone else if that feels right. If you wish, and if you have the energy, sort through your various possibilities as a way of setting your priorities and making up your mind.

Be living, not dying.

LAO TZU

Not life, but good life, is to be chiefly valued.

SOCRATES

If I knew the world were coming to an end tomorrow,
I would still go out
and plant my three apple trees today.

MARTIN LUTHER

- *Don't put off making your plans or carrying them out.* Time will not wait. Neither should you.

- *Don't let your life become too hectic.* Pace yourself. Don't push so hard that you compromise your health. Do one thing at a time. Give yourself the freedom to enjoy what you're choosing to do.

- *Stay flexible.* Many unknowns lie ahead of you. Go into this time with an open mind, ready to adapt. Do the best you can, but always be gentle with yourself.

- *Set short term goals.* Concentrate on accomplishing them. Then add more later if you feel like it.

- *More than anything else, stay in the present.* Fill completely the moments you're given. Breathe deeply. See vividly. Touch lovingly. Concentrate on *being* every bit as much as on *doing.* Better yet, concentrate on it more.

Through it all, *live* your dying. Live with all the gusto you can. Live with your heart flung open and your arms spread wide. Live as if there were no tomorrow. Then tomorrow, with your whole being, live that way again. ◪

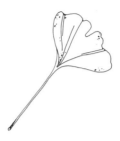

One cannot die hidden from God.

ITALIAN PROVERB

Lord, one day I will live with you
where you are.
May you live with me
where I am now.

JOHN MASON NEALE

11

Nurture yourself spiritually.

Whether or not you've had an active life of the soul, this can be a vital time for you spiritually. You now have a perspective you've never had before. Now you have an opportunity you'll never have again.

• *Nurturing yourself spiritually requires your time and your intention.* You must decide to give attention to this part of your life if you're to do it. It will not happen automatically just because you know death is approaching. You're the only one who can set aside the time this nurturing takes. Perhaps you'll want to inform others of your intention, or maybe writing it in your own heart is enough. Results are more likely and more effective if you make this a familiar practice. That does not mean, however, that this must be a labor for you. Make it a priority in your life, but don't make it a pain. Relax into the possibilities of what can happen.

• *Quiet helps.* It's difficult to access your soul without first stilling your mind. Often silence will assist you. So will peaceful music, or quiet sounds from nature, or the soothing voice of another. If you can create these tranquil interludes yourself, do so. If you need others' assistance in creating these times, be specific about what you'd like and what they can do to help.

• *You may turn to formal religious practices, or you may choose other means.* Your religious faith may have long served as a foundation for your life, in which case it's more likely to be a guide and comfort for you today. Your faith may be in a state of flux or upheaval, as you grapple with the strange new realities of your life. You may be one who has preferred to express your spirituality in less

*The most beautiful thing we can experience
is the mysterious.*

ALBERT EINSTEIN

May the Great Mystery make sunrise in your heart.

SIOUX PRAYER

*What it is that dwelleth here I know not,
yet my heart is full of awe
and the tears trickle down.*

SAIGYO

structured but no less meaningful ways. Do what works best for you. Remember, for example, that prayers can take many forms—they can be spoken or sung or read or listened to. Silent meditation may be its own eloquent prayer. Spiritual music, inspirational readings, religious symbols, and thoughtful rituals all have their place. Experiment for yourself.

• *Include others in this nurturing if you wish.* If it feels right, talk with another or others about the spiritual aspects of this journey you're on. Turn to a clergyperson or spiritual friend if you want. Pray with others or for others. Share in exercises of the soul with those you're close to spiritually. Allow those you trust to demonstrate their caring for you in this deep way.

• *Expect the unexpected.* You cannot always predict what experiences of spirituality will hold for you. You may grow calm as you express your innermost longings. Or you may go through a time of unrest or distress before that calm arrives. Sometimes dying people have experiences they cannot easily explain—intuitions, or voices, or visions. If that happens, don't be alarmed. Know that others before you have experienced something similar. Learn what there is to learn. See what you can see. Stay open.

What you may find most unexpected is how remarkable this experience can be. When your distractions are fewer, your powers of concentration can become greater. While your energy may recede, your passion can grow. While your questions may not all have answers, you can also discover they don't have to. Even if you cannot completely understand what awaits you, you can still do what we're all called to do—live our way into that mystery. And what an incredible way of living it can be! ◩

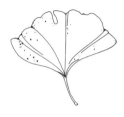

Hope is patience with the lamp lit.

TERTULLIAN

There never was night that had no morn.

DINAH MULOCK CRAIG

When God shuts a door,
God opens a window.

JOHN RUSKIN

12

Dare to hope.

You may have felt your life lost all hope when you received the news you had a terminal illness. You may feel that way still. Your days may seem sad and heavy, your nights long and scary. Your future may look bleak.

Feelings like these are understandable. If you have enjoyed life and loved others, such feelings are almost unavoidable, at least for awhile. No one likes giving up what brings pleasure. But the darker feelings you may experience need not have the final word. Other possibilities exist. You can dare to hope. And you can use whatever energy is at hand to turn some of those hopes into realities.

You may already be hoping that you'll experience only minimal physical discomfort as the days unfold. If that's true, you would do well to discuss pain control with your caregivers. You may hope to maintain your dignity as best you can throughout the time ahead. You may have specific hopes about where you'll spend your closing days, and how you'll spend them, and with whom. You may hope to die at a preferred time or in a preferred way. And, yes, you may even hope to live for a long, long time—sometimes that happens.

You may harbor other kinds of hopes—for instance, that this will be a time of inner healing. You may wish for release from past deeds or old wounds, from painful inadequacies or hurtful thoughts. You may wish to gain whatever benefits you can from looking at your life in its wholeness or from appreciating it for its richness. You may set your hopes on eventually achieving inner peace and outer calm. You

A death blow is a life blow to some
Who till they died, did not alive become;
Who had they lived, had died but when
They died, Vitality begun.

EMILY DICKINSON

You will go out in joy and be led forth in peace;
the mountains and hills before you will burst into song,
and all the trees of the field will clap their hands.

THE BOOK OF ISAIAH

may desire to make new discoveries as long as you draw breath, and even afterwards.

Perhaps you'll carry hopes for the kind of healing that involves others—not just that you can forgive another, for instance, but that another will forgive you. You may hold out for the possibility that this experience will draw you closer to those you love, and that they may draw closer to one another.

You may hope this can be a time of growth *for* other people as well as *with* other people. Your hope may be that your caregivers experience the sacredness of their work, and that your loved ones understand the delightfulness of their affection. Perhaps those around you can use this time to become less fearful of death and more open to life. Perhaps they can find joy in the midst of what now brings them sorrow. Perhaps they can learn from what you now have to teach.

Your hopes may take ever so many forms—that the time before you will be rich in meaning, that the journey ahead of you will be graceful in its transition, that the life awaiting you will be generous in its rewards. At some deep level you may hope that when your days on earth draw to a close, you will feel that your life has mattered, your love has been returned, your legacy has been assured, and your purpose has been fulfilled.

You have many possibilities, and they all begin with hope. ◪

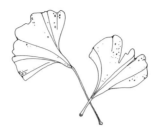

Destiny is not a matter of chance,
it is a matter of choice;
it is not a thing to be waited for,
it is a thing to be achieved.

WILLIAM JENNINGS BRYAN

Wherever your life ends, it is all there.
The advantage of living is not measured by length,
but by use;
some people have lived long and lived little;
attend to it while you are in it.
It lies in your will, not in the number of years,
for you have lived enough.

MICHEL DE MONTAIGNE

A Final Note

Yours is an unusual situation. You're the same person you've always been, but life is not the way it used to be. It's changed and it will remain changed.

You experience the same emotions you've always felt. But you feel them a little differently now. Sometimes there's an intensity you don't quite expect. Sometimes there's an urgency you can't quite predict. Sometimes a feeling may suddenly take your breath away.

Many things remain unchanged about the people who make up your life. They don't love you any less. If anything, they may love you even more. But a subtle change is occurring in how they relate to you. They're moving in one direction and you're glancing toward another. They know it, and so do you.

In the most essential way, you're no different than you were a month ago or a year ago. Yet in one inescapable way, you *are* different. Deep within, you are coming to grips with an unavoidable truth: your life no longer appears as unlimited as it once did. An end is in sight.

Another truth is just as real: you are no different from anyone else who lives today. The very same life surges through you as surges through them. And the very same death calls their name as surely as it calls yours. It's just that you hear the call more clearly, more closely. And once you hear the call, you cannot ignore it, nor can you forget it.

A question accompanies that call: "What will you do with what you now know?" Contrary to what others may say, contrary to what

God, grant me the serenity
to accept the things I cannot change,
the courage to change the things I can,
and the wisdom to know the difference.
Grant me patience with the things that take time,
tolerance of the struggles of others
that may be different from my own,
appreciation for all I have,
and the willingness to get up and try again,
one day at a time.

THE SERENITY PRAYER

you may think, you are not helpless in the face of all that is happening. There are choices you can make. You can still have a say in what your future holds for you.

• *You can choose to treat the time you're given however you wish.* You can see it as holding a promising opportunity or an inevitable duty. If you want, you can make the most of whatever your life still holds. You can fill as many of your moments as you can doing what you enjoy doing, being the way you enjoy being. You can use your eyes to really see, and your ears to really hear, and your fingers to really touch—maybe even for the first time. You can practice being as fully present as you know how. If it's important, you can try accomplishing what's within reason, and—who knows?—maybe even what's beyond reason.

• *You can respond within yourself however you will.* Whatever is happening to you, no one can dictate what will happen inside you. You are free to create your own attitudes. You may accentuate either one: the negative or the positive. You may repeat to yourself, "All is sadness." Or you may say to yourself, "Let's go find the joy." You may question "Why?" or you may admit "Why not?". You may ask yourself, "What am I supposed to learn here?". You may challenge yourself, "Where are the ways I can grow?".

• *You can relate to those around you however you choose.* You can treat them as you'd like to be treated, or some other way. You can reach out to them hoping they'll reach back to you, or you can pull away. It's within your power to speak openly and listen thoughtfully, or not. In your own unique way, you can care for those who care for you. You can cherish those who love you. You can hold those who'll miss you.

There is nothing I can give you which you do not have.

But there is much, very much,

that while I cannot give it, you can take.

No heaven can come to us unless our hearts

find rest in today.

Take heaven!

No peace lies in the future which is not hidden

in the present instant.

Take peace!

The gloom of the world is but a shadow.

Behind it, yet within reach, is joy.

There is a radiance and glory in the darkness,

could we but see,

and to see, we have only to look.

I beseech you to look.

FRA GIOVANNI

• *You can open yourself to the mystery that surrounds you.* You can explore the marvels that lie everywhere around you, both those you understand and those you don't. You can bare yourself to that miracle called life and that greater miracle called life beyond life. You can open yourself to the greatest Mystery of all—the One who has many names but only one essence, many faces but only one Love.

The poet Rabindranath Tagore once composed these words:

> *Let your life lightly dance on the edges of time*
> *like dew on the tip of a leaf.*

His words are worth repeating.

Let your life dance lightly on the edge of this time and on the edge of the time to come. Let it dance lightly with those you love, and with those who love you, and with all those who have *ever* loved you. Let it dance as long as it will and wherever it will and in the way that it will. Let your life lightly dance for all to see today and for all to remember tomorrow.

May your dance be the dance of a lifetime. And beyond. ◩

Additional Resources by James E. Miller

Illness, Dying, and Caregiving

Books

One You Love Is Dying
    12 Thoughts to Guide You on the Journey

When You're Ill or Incapacitated
    12 Things to Remember in Times of Sickness, Injury, or Disability
When You're the Caregiver
    12 Things to Do If Someone You Care For Is Ill or Incapacitated

The Caregiver's Book
    Caring for Another, Caring for Yourself

Welcoming Change
    Discovering Hope in Life's Transitions

A Pilgrimage Through Grief
    Healing the Soul's Hurt After Loss

Videotapes

The Grit and Grace of Being a Caregiver
    Maintaining Your Balance as You Care for Others

Listen to Your Sadness
    Finding Hope Again After Despair Invades Your Life

How Do I Go On?
    Re-designing Your Future After Crisis Has Changed Your Life

By the Waters of Babylon
    A Spiritual Pilgrimage for Those Who Feel Dislocated

The Natural Way of Prayer
    Being Free to Express What You Feel Deep Within

You Shall Not Be Overcome
    Promises and Prayers for Uncertain Times

Audiotapes

When You're Ill or Incapacitated
    12 Things to Remember in Times of Sickness, Injury, or Disability

Loss and Grief

Books

What Will Help Me?
12 Things to Remember When You Have Suffered a Loss
How Can I Help?
12 Things to Do When Someone You Know Suffers a Loss

Winter Grief, Summer Grace: *Returning to Life After a Loved One Dies*

How Will I Get Through the Holidays?
12 Ideas for Those Whose Loved One Has Died

Videotapes

Invincible Summer: *Returning to Life After Someone You Love Has Died*

We Will Remember: *A Meditation for Those Who Live On*

Nothing Is Permanent Except Change
Learning to Manage Transition in Your Life

Audiotapes

The Transforming Potential of Your Grief: *Eight Principles for Renewed Life*

Spirituality

Books

Autumn Wisdom: *Finding Meaning in Life's Later Years*

A Little Book for Preachers: *101 Ideas for Better Sermons*

Videotapes

Gaining a Heart of Wisdom: *Finding Meaning in the Autumn of Your Life*

Common Bushes Afire: *Discovering the Sacred in Our Everyday lives*

Why Yellow? *A Quiet Search for That Which Lies Behind All That Is*

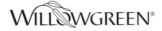

WILLOWGREEN®
P.O. Box 25180 • Fort Wayne, IN 46825 • 219/424-7916

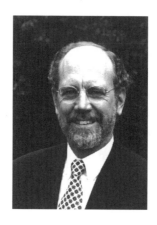

James E. Miller is a clergyman, grief counselor, writer, and photographer who lives and works in Fort Wayne, Indiana. Many of his books, audiotapes, and videotapes deal with illness, caregiving, loss, and grief, but his writing and photography also incorporate the topics of managing transition, healthy older age, and spirituality. He lectures and leads workshops widely, often utilizing his personal photography to illustrate his ideas. He is married to Bernie and together they have three children.

For information about his other resources, including quantity purchases, as well as about scheduling him for a speaking engagement or workshop, contact

Willowgreen
P.O. Box 25180
Fort Wayne, IN 46825
219/424-7916
jmiller@willowgreen.com